THE
BREAST PUMPING
WHISPERER

A Mother's Guide to Successful Breast Pumping

ABIGAEL MAXWELL, MD, FAAP

ISBN 13: 978-1946629-40-1
ISBN 10: 1-946629-40-5

TABLE OF CONTENTS

Testimonials

"The Breast Pumping Whisperer is a unique library addition and offers a variety of information for parents interested in the many aspects of providing breast milk for their babies. La Leche League USA encourages parents to include this guide as they seek support and educate themselves from as many diverse resources as there are [breastfeeding] families."

LLL USA
www.lllusa.org

The Breast Pumping Whisperer is a great resource for women who are pumping breast milk for their babies. With today's hectic life schedule, many women cannot stay home with their babies but must incorporate breastfeeding with working and pumping. Others may choose to exclusively pump and bottle feed. Abigael addresses both situations from the type of pump to use, to pumping schedules, traveling, and finally weaning. She's done it all herself and reports back to us on how you can do it too!

Julie Bouchet-Horwitz, FNP, IBCLC
Executive Director
The New York Milk Bank
Member of HMBANA

Dr. Abigael Maxwell is a mother, neonatologist, and a breastfeeding advocate. Her book **The Breast Pumping Whisperer: A Mother's Guide to Successful Breast Pumping** *is a much needed guide for every woman who is expecting or just had a baby and for every provider who is supporting women in their quest to breastfeed. The style of the book is personable and stems from the extensive experience of Dr. Maxwell successfully pumping exclusively to provide breast milk for her five children while pursuing her professional career. I particularly like the chapters where Dr. Maxwell reviews various breast pumps and provides sample schedules for pumping.*

Boriana Parvez, MD, IBCLC, Attending Neonatologist, Associate Director of the Neonatal Perinatal Fellowship Program, Medical Director, The Liquid Gold Preterm Milk Bank, Maria Fareri Children's Hospital, Westchester Medical Center, Valhalla, NY

The Breast Pumping Whisperer: A Mother's Guide to Successful Breast Pumping *is a must-read for new moms! Abigael Maxwell shares her experiences with pumping to provide breast milk for five of her own children and provides an excellent resource for mothers who want their babies to have the best start possible through proper nutrition. I highly recommend you not just read this book, but gift it to every expectant mother you know!*

Michelle Prince
Best-selling Author, Speaker, and Publisher
www.MichellePrince.com

Dr. Maxwell is such an inspiration and a fountain of wisdom, and her book The Breast Pumping Whisperer *is a true testament to that. It is filled with knowledge that a mother should have on every aspect of breastfeeding, from beginning to end. It is also an ultimate guide to any challenges and obstacles a mother could face throughout her breast pumping journey. This book is a must-read for every mom!*

Giselle Carlotta-McDonald, MPH

I have known Abigael for over ten years, and she has truly taken the art of breastfeeding to another level. Her practical tips, seasoned with applied wisdom, will help any mother in her breastfeeding journey. The Breast Pumping Whisperer *is a real keeper!*

Maua Mosha Alleyne, MPH and mom of three

Dr. Maxwell's book is a must-have resource for all working moms—mothers who work in the home or outside of the home. Her practical advice on sustaining or improving milk production is easy to understand and implement. Because of her book, I was able to establish a strong and consistent lactation schedule for both of my children, especially when I returned to work as an education professional.

Nicole Hughes, BA, Yale University; MST, Pace University; M.Ed, Columbia University, Campus Principal, Buchtel Community Learning Center

The Breast Pumping Whisperer is an informative, practical guide for all moms, but it is particularly refreshing for moms who have full careers outside the home and those with travel intensive careers. Often, moms like us think breastfeeding is out of our grasp and wonder how we can reconcile our desire to give our babies nutrient-rich breast milk with our challenging schedules. Dr. Maxwell simplifies an expansive topic—breastfeeding—and gives troubleshooting advice on how to pump in an airport, how to recruit your partner as a critical member in this experience, get milk through airport security, increase supply, and store milk while away in hotels. As a career mom of two who breastfed and pumped in many circumstances, I appreciate how accessible Dr. Maxwell makes breast pumping. Where there is a will, there is a way! Empowering and caring medical professionals like her are why I was able to give breast milk to my two children, one of whom has a rare disease, for over a year. It has been a key factor in their positive health outcomes!

Anna Blanding Pilliner, BA Yale University,
MBA Yale School of Management
Owner, The Pilliner Group
Hamden, CT and mom of two

We know that breast pumping has become an essential part of breastfeeding in that many mothers return to work and/or find they cannot be with their babies at every feeding. However, not every mother knows how to meet her breastfeeding goals with the aid of a breast pump. In this informative and highly practical book, Abigael Maxwell explains in detail how to maintain your milk supply with a breast pump through her personal experience and expertise. She also uses real stories about the challenges she faced! This is a must read book for moms who anticipate the need for breast pumping!

Rhonda Valdes-Greene RN, MSN, IBCLC

INTRODUCTION

I am excited about breastfeeding! I love to see when a new mom and her baby get their breastfeeding rhythm and the confidence that emanates from the mother when she realizes she can feed her baby well. Personally, I have made the journey myself five times with my children. I have to admit, I did not have any in-depth conversations with my OB or my future pediatrician about breastfeeding. We attended a Lamaze course over the span of six weeks, and they barely mentioned breastfeeding. As a matter of fact, my husband was advised by a co-worker that I should get a breast pump before our first child was born. Figuring out how to use the pieces was interesting! Due to my busy schedule (I was in medical school), I opted to use a breast pump so my husband and in-laws could help to take care of our first baby while I studied for exams.

I have to give a special shout out to friends who gave me practical hands-on advice on using the breast pump. They were truly my go-to guides for different hiccups I had along the way with low supply after traveling and how to store the breast milk. Since then, I have had four more children, and I have not only grown in my confidence with providing breast milk for each one of my babies, but I have also become a resource to my friends who subsequently had babies and questions on how to breastfeed. I would like to thank my family for their patience and support through this journey, and finally, I am indebted to my husband, Kerry, who recognized and pulled this book out of me even when I doubted myself. Thank you!

So it is with this joy and experience that I am paying it forward to be a resource to YOU and so many other moms. I want to empower women and those who care for babies to be advocates for ideal nutrition for infants. I'm excited about helping you on your journey. Let's begin!

Now this book is not necessarily a "how-to" breastfeed book—in other words, I won't be discussing the various techniques with feeding from the breast itself. For any issues surrounding that, I recommend you talk to your physician or a lactation consultant.

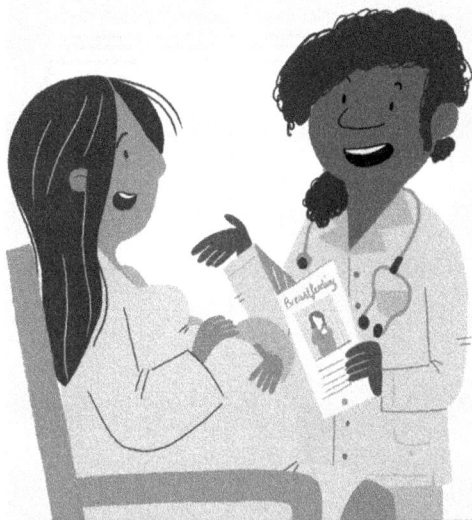

BREASTFEEDING SUPPORT — World Health Organization — unicef

BEFORE YOUR BABY IS BORN

YOUR HEALTH WORKER IS THERE TO

TALK WITH YOU ABOUT HOW YOU PLAN TO FEED YOUR BABY.

EXPLAIN THE BENEFITS OF BREASTFEEDING FOR YOU AND YOUR BABY.

SUPPORT YOU TO TRY AGAIN IF YOU DIDN'T BREASTFEED YOUR FIRST BABY.

MOST WOMEN ARE ABLE TO BREASTFEED WITH THE RIGHT SUPPORT.

CHAPTER 1

AFFIRMATION TO MOTHERS WHO CANNOT/CHOOSE NOT TO BREASTFEED

I would like to start this book by affirming those moms who cannot or choose not to breastfeed their babies. This is obviously a personal decision. This book is specifically written for those mothers who choose to breastfeed. It will help them along that journey (and it is definitely a journey and not a sprint). It is also intended for mothers who are revisiting breastfeeding after a failed attempt in a prior pregnancy. Just because it didn't work for you last time doesn't exclude you from trying again!

It is my goal to empower women in this journey and to point them to the adequate resources.

CHAPTER 2

BENEFITS OF BREAST MILK TO YOUR BABY

I can rattle off the numerous benefits of breast milk to your baby, as I'm sure you can. They include decreased incidence of ear infections in the first year of life, decreased incidence of childhood asthma, decreased viral URIs, and obesity. But did you know that breast milk is full of antiviral and antibacterial properties such as interleukins and cytokines as well as growth factors. Our bodies adapt to the gestational age that our babies are born, and the content of the milk varies depending on how far along in your pregnancy you were when your baby was born and how old your baby currently is.

Let me break this down. If your baby is born at 7 months of pregnancy (28-31 weeks), then that milk is much higher in protein, fat, and antibacterial properties than breast milk for a baby who is born at 9 months of pregnancy. Furthermore, the milk that your body produces in the first week of your baby's life is also different in composition from the milk that your body produces at four weeks after birth. Why do I say this?

Breast milk is a dynamic food! Our bodies adapt the composition of it depending on the time of birth as well as what is going on with the mother. (If mom has a cold, for example, her breast milk will contain more interleukins.)

There is also a decreased incidence of milk intolerance. As a matter of fact, for babies who have short gut (more often seen in extremely premature babies), they oftentimes cannot tolerate regular formula and the protein composition in it. Breast milk is usually the preferred nutrition (whether it is mom's milk or donor milk) over formula.

So why should I give my baby breast milk? Well, the number one reason is that our babies were designed to ingest human milk for nutrition. Simple as that.

Let's face it—the beginning matters. I think we can all agree on the importance of good nutrition for a baby before, during, and even after pregnancy—and why is that? A woman needs to create the optimal environment for her baby to develop and grow, and that goes for after the baby is born, as well. The nutrients that will be derived from the breast milk are all nutrients that are or are not in your body. Breast milk is not only a "first food" but also nutrition for your baby.

I'll be the first to admit that we as physicians are not always the best advocates for breastfeeding (particularly obstetricians, family medicine, pediatricians, and other providers who care for pregnant women and, subsequently, their infants). Part of it could be that we might not have a level of comfort when speaking about breastfeeding. However, in spite of having or not having a conversation with your healthcare provider about breastfeeding, mothers can still equip themselves with the information and support needed to have a successful breastfeeding experience.

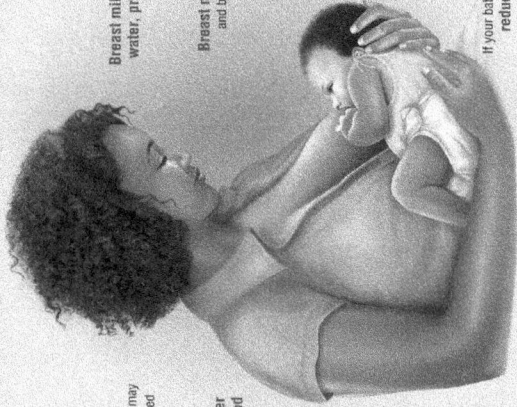

Breastfeeding Benefits

For Baby

Breast milk has the right amount of fat, sugar, water, protein, and minerals needed for a baby's growth and development.

Breast milk is easier to digest than formula, and breastfed babies have less gas, fewer feeding problems, and less constipation.

Breast milk contains antibodies that protect infants from certain illnesses, such as ear infections, diarrhea, respiratory illnesses, and allergies.

Breastfed infants have a lower risk of sudden infant death syndrome.

If your baby is born preterm, breast milk can help reduce the risk of many of the short-term and long-term health problems.

For Mom

Breastfeeding burns as many as 500 extra calories each day, which may make it easier to lose the weight you gained during pregnancy.

Women who breastfed longer have lower rates of type 2 diabetes, high blood pressure, and heart disease.

Women who breastfed have lower rates of breast cancer and ovarian cancer.

Breastfeeding triggers the release of oxytocin that causes the uterus to contract and may decrease the amount of bleeding you have after giving birth.

For additional information and resources,
go to www.aaog.org/breastfeeding

The American College of
Obstetricians and Gynecologists
WOMEN'S HEALTH CARE PHYSICIANS

CHAPTER 3

BENEFITS OF BREASTFEEDING TO MOM

Oftentimes, we don't explore the benefits of breastfeeding to mom, and boy, there are plenty! Health benefits range from a decrease in overall risk of ovarian, breast, and uterine cancer to more rapid weight loss.

There is increased flexibility particularly if you choose to use a breast pump. This allows other family members and loved ones to participate in feeding your baby and giving you some time to do other things or even get more rest! Having a supportive home environment will greatly aid in this process, and a supportive family can also participate in helping to wash the bottles and other breast pumping equipment, getting you some water or juice while you are breastfeeding or pumping, and minimizing other distractions during feeding or pumping time. You can also get more sleep, particularly at night, if your partner gets up to feed the baby while you are using the breast pump. They can feed and bond with baby while you use the pump and go back to bed. (And which new mom doesn't want more sleep?)

So I know you might be thinking "How can using the breast pump really save me time?" Well, let's look at time in the short term and in the long term. If you pump 8-12 times a day and for 20 minutes on average, you'll spend anywhere between 160-240 minutes (2.5 to 4 hours) using the breast pump. You can create a more predictable schedule for yourself and your baby. If you were to breastfeed, on the other hand, the time that your baby is attached to you is highly variable.

I believe that when it comes to rearing children, we have to have the long goal in mind. If I ask a room of 100 parents "Who wants the best for your child?" I guarantee that all 100 will raise their hands! And if any parent does not raise their hand, it's probably due to shyness. I believe that conversations around breastfeeding have become so polarized that many people tiptoe around it and are afraid to offend the pro-breastfeeding moms and the pro-formula feeding moms. This is no competition! As I stated previously in my introduction, this book is written for women who are thinking about breastfeeding (in hopes that I can convince you to choose to breastfeed your baby) and for those who have decided to breastfeed. I believe with adequate resources, moms will be even more empowered in their decision.

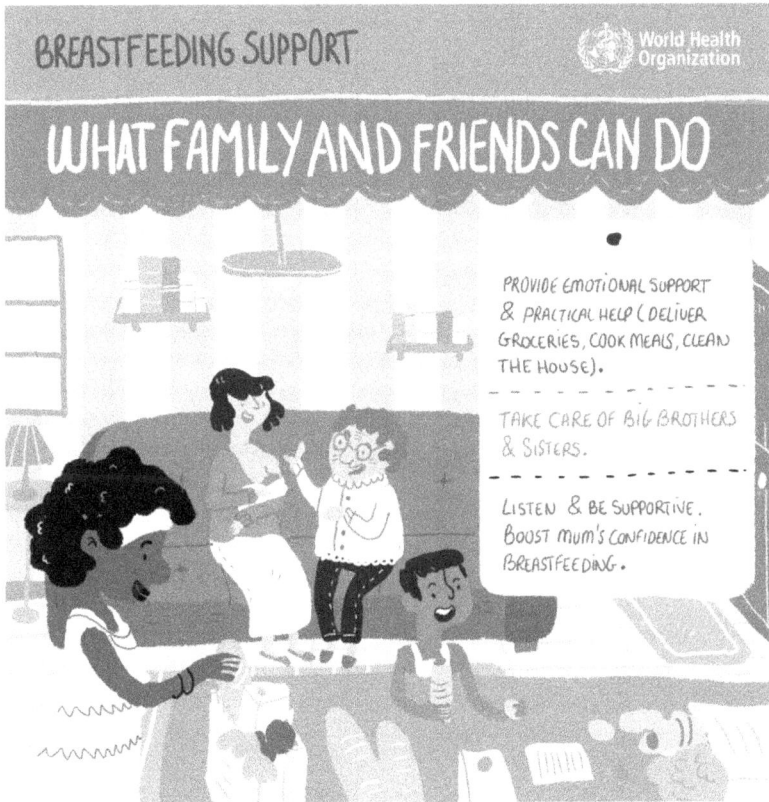

BREASTFEEDING SUPPORT

World Health Organization

WHAT FAMILY AND FRIENDS CAN DO

PROVIDE EMOTIONAL SUPPORT & PRACTICAL HELP (DELIVER GROCERIES, COOK MEALS, CLEAN THE HOUSE).

TAKE CARE OF BIG BROTHERS & SISTERS.

LISTEN & BE SUPPORTIVE. BOOST MUM'S CONFIDENCE IN BREASTFEEDING.

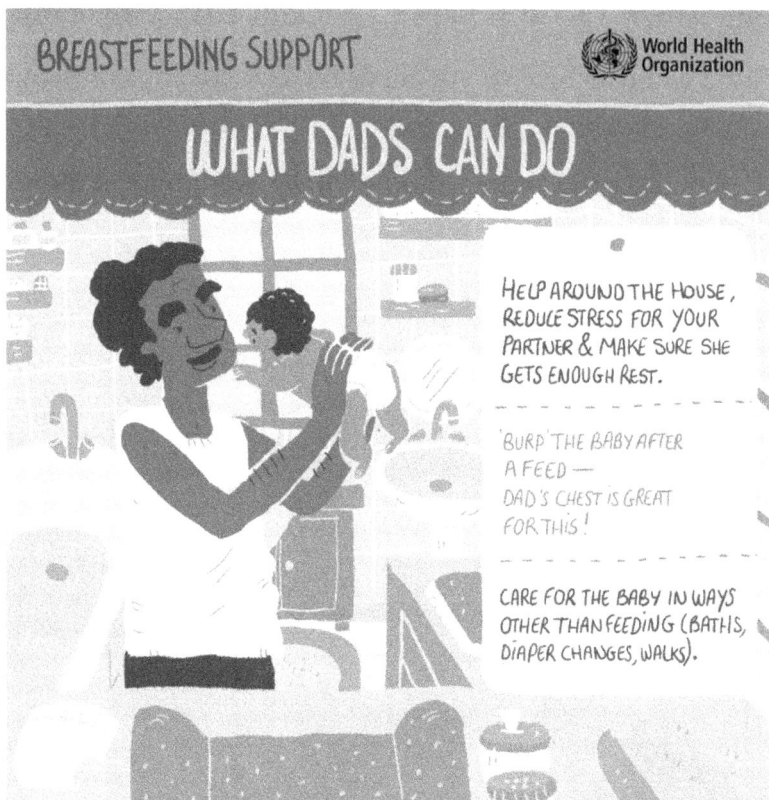

Now, for some moms, they may be the first living women in their families to breastfeed. You might even get pushback from your relatives on your decision. This is a perfect opportunity to respectfully let them know that this is a decision you have decided to make for your baby, and then you can share with them how they can be supportive. Most families are eager to help a new parent, and hopefully your family falls in this category!

CHAPTER 4

HAND EXPRESSION OF COLOSTRUM

Colostrum is the fluid produced by the breasts immediately after giving birth. It is nutrient rich and loaded with immune, growth, tissue, and repair factors. It aids in the development of the immunity in newborns. Studies have demonstrated that a woman can increase her milk supply significantly by initiating hand expression within the first few hours after birth, particularly if her baby is born pre-term or too sick to breastfeed directly. I have personally experienced that my milk supply came in sooner after hand expressing. Some women also hand express after using the breast pump to remove any residual milk from their breasts. Over time, this leads to an increase in milk production.

There is a video on the following website that demonstrates how to express colostrum. It's an older video, but the content is very useful. You can find it on the Stanford Medicine website (search for hand expression of breast milk).

There is also a video at https://vimeo.com/65196007 that demonstrates how to massage your breasts to initiate milk let down, and it explains hand expression of colostrum and milk. The key is to remember that light massage works better than a more aggressive massage. The more frequently milk is expressed, the sooner the milk comes in and the more milk is produced.

CHAPTER 5

WHEN SHOULD I NOT BREASTFEED?

There are certain conditions under which a mom should either not breastfeed directly from the breast or not give expressed breast milk to the baby. Certainly, if a woman is undergoing chemotherapy or radiation, providing breast milk is contraindicated (strongly not recommended). Also, if a mom has HSV (Herpes Simplex Virus) of the breast or nipple, she should not breastfeed until it clears up. Untreated tuberculosis is also a contraindication to breastfeeding (until mom starts anti-microbial therapy).

If mom has a simple infection such as a UTI, viral upper respiratory tract infection, skin infection, etc., then she can continue to breastfeed. As a matter of fact, the breast milk might actually look different in color during and shortly after illness, and this is perfectly normal. Some women describe the breast milk as being more orange or yellow.

If a mom has a serious infection that leads to sepsis, she may continue to use the breast pump, but it is recommended that the milk be dumped (i.e., pump and dump). Only after she has repeated negative blood cultures can she resume giving the baby the breast milk. (For example, if Monica has a positive blood infection on January 3, she should continue to use the breast pump and discard her milk. If the repeat blood culture on January 5 is negative, then any milk pumped after January 5 can be given to her baby).

In addition to chemotherapy, there are also certain medications that have an increased risk of being present in the breast milk (especially if the medication is highly lipophilic (i.e., fat loving and therefore potentially harmful to your baby). I will not provide an exhaustive list of these medications in this book; however, I will provide a few types of medications, including anti-seizure medications and certain psychotic medications. (If you are on these medications, do NOT stop taking them as the benefit of the medication to you as a mother outweighs the benefit of stopping so you can breastfeed your baby). A useful reference that I use for mothers of my patients is LactMed.org. Now just to give you a heads up, the resource oftentimes will not give conclusive advice on whether to breastfeed or not, or if you should provide expressed breast milk if ingesting certain medications. Thus, I always recommend discussing this with either your healthcare provider or the healthcare provider for your baby.

Certainly, if you use/abuse prescription medications and/or illicit drugs, I strongly advise that you seek professional help in stopping, and in the meantime, given the transference of these drugs to the baby in variable amounts in the breast milk, I would recommend against breastfeeding or giving your baby your expressed breast milk.

CHAPTER 6

GETTING OVER THE FEAR OF USING A BOTTLE

First, let me start by saying "It's PERFECTLY okay to use a bottle!!" I know mothers might get conflicting messages about when to introduce a bottle if they want to exclusively breastfeed. They wonder if it will cause nipple confusion and if they should spoon feed or use other methods of feeding.

My answer is KEEP IT SIMPLE!! I cannot count the number of moms who have been stressed or left confused about breastfeeding or using a bottle, and that has oftentimes turned them off from the entire idea of breastfeeding.

The first question to ask yourself is "What are my goals of breastfeeding? Is it to provide breast milk to my baby? Is it to bond through the process of actual breastfeeding?"

Sit and think about this. The answers will help inform your decision on breastfeeding

You might be the only person in your family to breast-feed—and that's OKAY.

So, take a deep breath and tell yourself "It's OKAY if I use a bottle for my baby." Now, even though I'm advocating using a bottle if needed, I'm still advocating for breast milk! It's only once we recognize and address our fears that we can move forward successfully.

CHAPTER 7

What to Do with Engorged Breasts

This is a common problem that moms experience, and it's usually due to breastfeeding sessions that were spaced too far apart. It also usually occurs a few days after delivery. Not only are engorged breasts painful for mom, they can also make breastfeeding challenging for your baby. First, you need to differentiate between engorged breasts (breasts may feel very firm or even hard, tender, etc.) versus mastitis. Due to an infection, breasts may also feel hard and tender. However, they will feel warm to the touch, and you might even have some reddened areas and a fever. If you do feel as if you have an infection, then you will need to see your healthcare provider.

Any mom who has had engorged breasts knows the immediate priority is RELIEF! Here are a few suggestions that have personally worked for me:

23

1. Before breastfeeding or breast pumping, **gently** massage the breasts in a circular fashion, starting from the outer breast and then moving inward towards the areola. Put warm compresses on for 3-5 minutes or take a quick hot shower. This softens the breasts and starts to get the milk flowing.

2. During the breastfeeding or breast pumping session, you can continue to gently massage your breasts.

3. After you have completed the breastfeeding or breast pumping session, apply cold compresses to your breasts for up to 10 minutes to reduce the swelling. You can also apply cold compresses in between feedings/pumping sessions for relief of swelling. Some moms put a cabbage leaf in the freezer and apply it to their breasts (in the bra) until it warms up. You can also use an ice pack. Once the breasts have softened, stay vigilant about the frequency of your breastfeeding sessions or breast pumping sessions. If your baby has taken a nap that is longer than normal, feel free to use the breast pump to empty your breasts.

To minimize discomfort while pumping, consider the following suggestions. If your nipples feel irritated or look red, make sure the flanges are the proper size because incorrectly sized flanges can lead to soreness, blocked milk ducts, and decreased milk production. (Most flanges range in size from 21 mm to 36 mm). To assess if your flange is the right size, ask the following questions during a breast pumping session:

1. Does your nipple move freely in the flange? The nipple should not rub against the flange.

2. How much areola tissue is being pulled into the flange tunnel? If there is no movement of the areola, the flange might be too small. If a large portion of your areola is being pulled into the tunnel, the flange is too big

3. Do you feel any discomfort or pain while pumping? If so, the flange is likely not fitting properly.

4. Do your breasts feel soft after using the breast pump?

5. Do you notice that your breasts are moving gently while pumping?

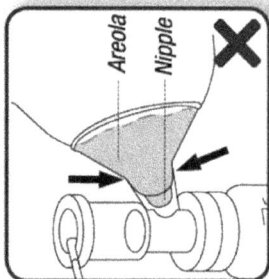

Good Fit

During pumping, your nipple moves freely in the breast flange tunnel. You see space around the nipple. Not much areola is drawn into the tunnel with the nipple.

Too Small

During pumping, some or all of your nipple rubs against the sides of the breast flange tunnel.

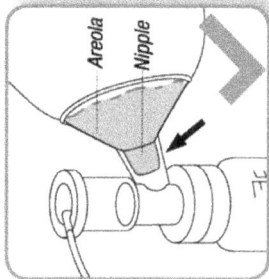

Too Large

During pumping, more areola is drawn into the breast flange with your nipple. Your areola may rub against the side of the breast flange tunnel.

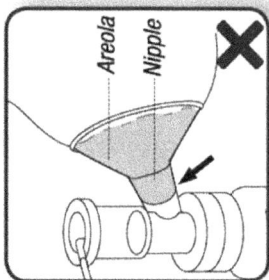

Image courtesy of Ameda Inc.

26

After ensuring the proper flange size, consider warming the flanges with hot water before pumping to optimize the sensation while pumping. Also use lanolin prior to pumping to minimize nipple irritation.

Also to minimize discomfort, start with low power and low frequency and gradually increase both when comfortable. When babies feed from the breast, they initially have a fast, less powerful suck, and then it becomes slow, rhythmic, and stronger. Adjust the pump cycle to find the most comfortable setting for you.

CHAPTER 8

BREAST PUMPING WHILE WORKING

This is one of the "ultimate challenges." You've been home with your baby for some time, and now it's time to return to the work environment. If you're like me, you probably have some anxiety surrounding this. But with a well thought-out plan, you'll transition to work in an efficient manner. First, speak with your employer/supervisor and let them know that you will need both time and a private, clean space to use the breast pump. Many offices and companies have designated breastfeeding/breast pumping rooms for mothers, and if you're fortunate to work for one of those companies, take full advantage. I've personally had to pump in my vehicle at times if a private space was not available.

Once you let the relevant people know about your intentions to breastfeed, start to think about your pumping schedule. So if your baby feeds about 8 times in a 24-hour period and you work 9 to 5, you can plan on using the breast pump at least 3 times while at work. Remember, you have the right to breastfeed while at work. When you pack for work, bring extra water and the following supplies in addition to your breast pump—breast pads, coverall for privacy, and a cooler to store milk and snacks for yourself. You will oftentimes be pleasantly surprised at how many employers and fellow employees will support you in your decision to breastfeed. If you happen to have a not-so-enthusiastic employer or fellow employees, be encouraged! With careful planning, you usually will be able to carve out time to use the breast pump.

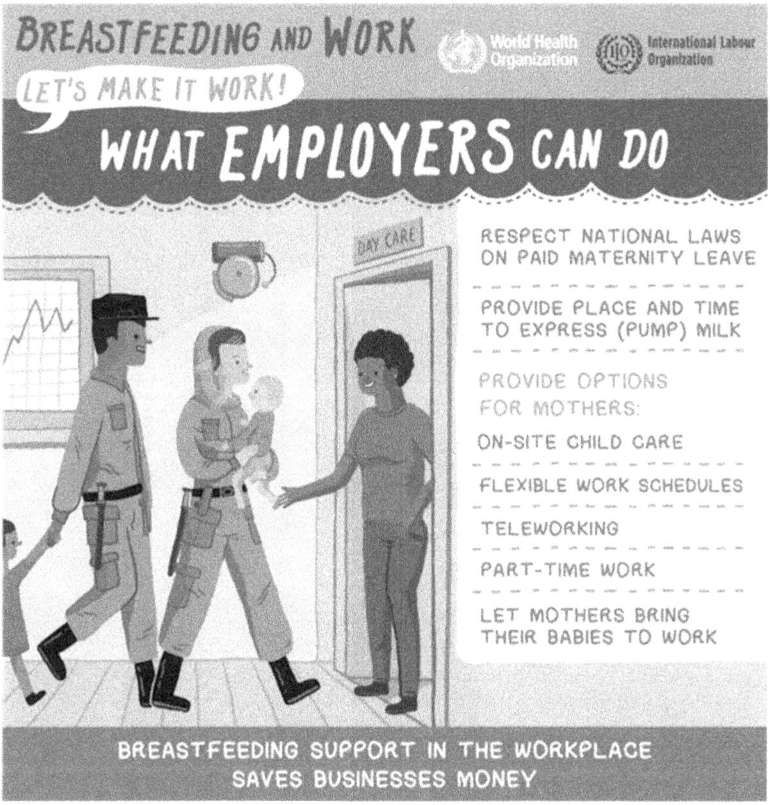
BREASTFEEDING AND WORK
World Health Organization
International Labour Organization
LET'S MAKE IT WORK!
WHAT EMPLOYERS CAN DO
DAY CARE
RESPECT NATIONAL LAWS ON PAID MATERNITY LEAVE
PROVIDE PLACE AND TIME TO EXPRESS (PUMP) MILK
PROVIDE OPTIONS FOR MOTHERS:
ON-SITE CHILD CARE
FLEXIBLE WORK SCHEDULES
TELEWORKING
PART-TIME WORK
LET MOTHERS BRING THEIR BABIES TO WORK
BREASTFEEDING SUPPORT IN THE WORKPLACE SAVES BUSINESSES MONEY

CHAPTER 9

BREAST PUMPING WHILE TRAVELING

"Where's your baby?"

Traveling with an infant (or without your baby, as is the case for many moms) definitely presents an interesting challenge to say the least. I vividly remember flying across the country when my baby was 4 months old with my breast pump and supplies in tow. I had already spoken with a few other friends who also traveled while breast-feeding, and they gave me their tips for streamlining the process. I even contacted TSA to confirm that there is no limit on how much milk I can bring with me.

Despite all this, I'll never forget a conversation I had at security in a major airport. I had several bags of expressed breast milk, and after putting them on the conveyer belt, I was pulled aside for additional questioning, which was nothing unusual. But this instance was unlike my other experiences. The TSA agent asked why I had so much milk, and I explained that I had traveled for a meeting and had to use a breast pump during my time away from my baby. Then he proceeds to ask me, "**Well, if you have so much milk, WHERE IS YOUR BABY?**"

This was a literal mic drop moment for me! I probably had to pick my jaw off the floor. I was honestly stunned and could not think of a response. All kinds of thoughts were running through my head, with the first one being "Is he really serious? Who asks that??" I had JUST explained that I was traveling home from a conference and had been away from my baby. After about 20 seconds, I got myself together and calmly said, "My baby is not with me—THAT'S the reason I am using a breast pump and why I have so much milk." He quickly realized the lack of depth of his question and told me I could collect the milk and continue to my gate.

So I'll start off by talking about breast pumping while in an airplane or airport. The good news is that many airports have now started to accommodate breastfeeding moms. Before traveling, you can call the airport to ask if they have designated spaces for you to use. I have even seen airports that have stand-alone breastfeeding pods in the hallway (Mamava). Other airports have rooms that have been re-designated and re-purposed for privacy and have sinks and comfortable couches for moms to sit in. However, not all airports are up to speed, so at times, you might have to be creative.

I would advise using the family bathroom or "companion care" bathroom, and if those are not available, use a handicap bathroom and clear off counter space to hold the pump. For flights over three to four hours long, I recommend pumping shortly before boarding the airplane so you can avoid at least one pumping session on the plane. For international travel, I would strongly advise searching online for the policies of the airports you will be traveling through. In general, most international airports will allow transport of breast milk through security, but be patient and prepare to explain why you have a breast pump and bags of breast milk.

I remember traveling in Ethiopia and putting my breast pump through the conveyer belt in security. I was pulled aside so the agent could investigate the pump. The agent actually tried to remove the motor from the breast pump (after which I promptly informed him that the motor is actually attached to the pump and cannot be removed). The model that I had at the time was an older one (in 2006), and I'm sure models now have motors that can be separated from the pump itself.

Also, be conscious of the type of electricity you will be using (alternating current or direct current). I would advise using your battery pack instead of a converter. (I used a converter in Ethiopia and ended up burning the breast pump motor.) I cannot overemphasize the importance of bringing extra batteries for your breast pump. When you are on the plane, you might have to pump right in your seat. Unfortunately, I have not seen any designated areas on the plane to pump aside from using the bathroom and placing your pump on the area designated for a changing table.

If you are wondering what supplies to bring with you while traveling, don't worry. I'll add a list at the end of this chapter. Depending on the length of your travels, you might want to ship frozen milk back home. For direct flights, I recommend checking in frozen milk with your suitcase. If you have a layover, I would advise bringing the frozen milk in a carry-on bag or cooler just in case there is a problem with the connecting flight. (You don't want the milk to get spoiled by being unrefrigerated for over 24 hours.)

Most cars also have adaptors for utilizing breast pumps in the vehicle. (Oftentimes, you can use the cigarette lighter.) Other cars have electrical outlets that can be used as well. Keep in mind that in order to achieve the same suction power while pumping in the vehicle, you might have to turn up the dial in the suction/power of the pump.

Low Supply

Unfortunately after traveling, your milk supply might decrease to an extent. Don't worry! Add a few extra breastfeeding sessions over the next 2-3 days, and you will be able to bring back your supply to what it was before you traveled. You can also power pump. (This imitates cluster feeding.) This involves sitting for an hour and pumping off and on during a one-hour interval. For example, you can pump for 10 minutes, then rest for 10 minutes (or pump for 20 minutes and rest for 10 minutes) and repeat again (twice in one hour). Do this at least twice a day for 2-3 days. You should experience milk letdown with the power pumping sessions and on overall an increase in milk supply.

Also, utilize hand expression after pumping as well as massaging your breasts before and during pumping to increase the milk supply. Some moms have also experienced that if they hold their babies more (especially skin to skin), it stimulates milk letdown.

Supplies to bring while traveling

- ☐ *Cooler (hard or soft, depending on the length of your travels -- a weekend versus a week or longer)*

- ☐ *Ice pack to transport fresh milk (Alternatively, if you will be bringing back frozen milk with you, you can put the fresh milk in the midst of the frozen milk.)*

- ☐ *Batteries for your battery pack*

- ☐ *Towel to wrap around frozen milk and place in cooler*

- ☐ *Milk storage bags*

- ☐ *Supplies to clean breast pump parts (i.e., bottle brush, dish soap, etc.)*

Accessible version: www.cdc.gov/healthywater/hygiene/healthychildcare/infantfeeding/breastpumps.html

How to Keep Your
Breast Pump Kit Clean

Providing breast milk is one of the best things you can do for your baby's health and development. Pumping your milk is one way to provide breast milk to your baby. Keeping the parts of your pump clean is critical, because germs can grow quickly in breast milk or breast milk residue that remains on pump parts. Following these steps can help prevent contamination and protect your baby from infection. If your baby was born prematurely or has other health concerns, your baby's health care providers may have more recommendations for pumping breast milk safely.

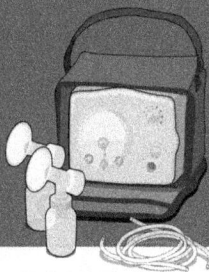

BEFORE EVERY USE

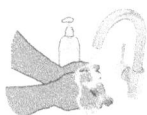

Wash hands with soap and water.

Inspect and assemble clean pump kit. If your tubing is moldy, discard and replace immediately.

Clean pump dials, power switch, and countertop with disinfectant wipes, especially if using a shared pump.

AFTER EVERY USE

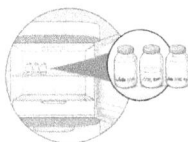

Store milk safely. Cap milk collection bottle or seal milk collection bag, label with date and time, and immediately place in a refrigerator, freezer, or cooler bag with ice packs.

Clean pumping area, especially if using a shared pump. Clean the dials, power switch, and countertop with disinfectant wipes.

Take apart breast pump tubing and separate all parts that come in contact with breast/breast milk.

Rinse breast pump parts that come into contact with breast/breast milk by holding under running water to remove remaining milk. Do not place parts in sink to rinse.

Clean pump parts that come into contact with breast/breast milk as soon as possible after pumping. You can clean your pump parts **in a dishwasher** or **by hand** in a wash basin used only for cleaning the pump kit and infant feeding items.

Follow the cleaning steps given on the next page.

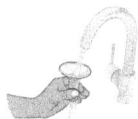

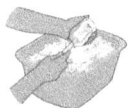

**Centers for Disease
Control and Prevention**
National Center for Emerging and
Zoonotic Infectious Diseases

CHAPTER 10

How to Increase Your Supply

"Basic Economics of Supply and Demand"

As an economics major in college, one of the basic tenets of the field is the rule of supply and demand—demand drives supply. It is as simple as that for breastfeeding as well. It is maintained by local feedback mechanisms (autocrine control). There really is no magic pill or special diet that will dramatically increase your supply. Now this excludes those mothers whose pituitary glands are unable to produce sufficient hormones for lactation (Sheehan's Syndrome).

Several factors play into increasing your milk supply, but for the sake of simplicity, I will break them down into two areas—diet and expression of milk. Let's start off with diet. First ensure that your water intake is adequate. Lactation consultants recommend drinking water frequently, preferably before you're thirsty, and to drink more if your urine appears dark yellow. Also, ensure that your diet is balanced and your calorie intake is sufficient. Generally, you need an additional 300-500 calories per day if your baby is receiving an exclusive breast milk diet. There are a few herbals that some women have attested to; however, before ingesting any of these, talk with your lactation consultant or healthcare provider to determine if these are appropriate for you. Certain foods are considered to be galactogogues (promote lactation). These include whole grains (oatmeal), dark leafy vegetables (kale, spinach), fennel, fenugreek, garlic, chickpeas, nuts (almonds), and ginger.

Expression of milk should start within the first hour after birth. Babies should either be allowed to latch onto the breast, or if your baby is unable to latch (due to being too sick or premature), hand expression should be initiated. To increase milk supply, after breastfeeding or breast pumping, hand express each breast for a total of 5 minutes to relieve the breast of any residual milk. (Reference the chapter "Hand Expression of Colostrum" for instructions on how to hand express your milk.) Pumping or breastfeeding every 2 hours for 3 days will also increase supply. You can also power pump. If the baby does not want to breastfeed, then you can hand express or use the breast pump to ensure that you have at least 12 breastfeeding occurrences in a 24-hour period. This will mean getting up to breast pump at night if your baby sleeps all night in order to empty your breasts. This will prompt the pituitary gland to produce more prolactin (which stimulates milk production). Be aware that your milk supply will often decrease after an illness, travel, or any other change to your normal routine.

In summary, lactating mothers who are experiencing a low milk supply should try to address this as a supply and demand response. Taking care of yourself seems like a cliché, but it essentially wraps up the approach—drinking enough fluids, getting adequate rest, breastfeeding in shorter intervals, or using the breast pump more often. Sometimes this might mean getting up at night to use the breast pump even if your baby is asleep. After a few days of this, you should see an increase in your supply and your baby more satisfied after feeding.

CHAPTER 11

WHAT TO DO
WITH OVERSUPPLY

There are some lactating women who have a problem with oversupply. This is a good problem to have! There are several ways to address this, ranging from how to decrease your milk supply to what to do with the excess breast milk (particularly for those women who are using the breast pump). You can donate to a milk bank (the milk is usually purchased for preterm babies or any infant who has an acute or chronic illness in which they do not tolerate formula), give it to a friend, sell it online (least preferred), or freeze the milk for later use (especially when your infant goes through a growth spurt and consumes more milk). Having an oversupply has also enabled some women to stop breastfeeding sooner than planned, and their infant still has milk to complete the 6-12 months of recommended breastfeeding duration.

If you are considering donating to a milk bank, you should familiarize yourself with the process. Human Milk Banking Association of North America (HMBANA) is the umbrella organization that oversees milk banks in the U.S. There are several questions that are asked, ranging from your country of birth, any recent travel, a list of medications that you ingest, any significant medical illnesses, and any past or current infections that will disqualify you from donating milk. This is to ensure the safety of the milk especially for the vulnerable population that it serves (usually preterm infants who have a compromised immune system). For those women who pass the initial screening, the mother's blood is tested for five infectious diseases. If the blood tests are negative, then the donated milk is processed. The milk is defrosted, pooled, pasteurized (pasteurization kills heat labile bacteria), and cultured to make sure it is free from harmful bacteria. There are a host of websites that serve as a platform for women to buy and sell breast milk. The price ranges vary. Keep in mind that these online sites are not regulated by any particular body, and a few independent studies have demonstrated that the milk sometimes is compromised (for example, someone might add other liquids to the breast milk to make it appear to be more than it actually is).

Other women might serve as "wet nurses" and provide breast milk informally to other women who are unable to provide adequate milk for their own babies. This is usually done without an exchange of monies. The mother whose infant will be receiving the donated milk understands that the milk is not tested, and therefore, there is always a potential risk of the infant getting sick. One common organism that infants can acquire from breast milk is CMV. This is usually fine in full term infants, but preterm infants might develop systemic illness from CMV that could have long-term consequences.

Some women address oversupply by either breast pumping less or breastfeeding less. Now, this method can lead to discomfort because the breasts can become engorged or develop mastitis, which would require antibiotics.

Last but not least, you can store extra breast milk in a freezer. It can last up to twelve months in a dedicated deep freezer. Once milk is thawed, it needs to be used within 24 hours and should not be rewarmed.

Whichever way you decide to address oversupply, know that there are several options.

CHAPTER 12

How to Wean from Breast Pumping

The decision to stop breastfeeding is a personal one, and the transition is better facilitated and tolerated (by both mom and infant) when it is planned in advance. For some mothers, there is an abundant supply of milk in the freezer that will allow her to still supply milk for her infant without having to pump any longer.

Weaning is usually done by slowly decreasing the number of sessions in which you use the breast pump. You can drop one breast pumping session every 2-3 days. Then when you're down to three breast pumping sessions a day, decrease the amount of time that you pump (so if you pump for 30 minutes, decrease the pumping time to 20 minutes) and continue for 2 days. Then drop a pumping session. Now you can pump every 12 hours for 2-3 days, then go down to pumping once a day. Continue to

ABIGAEL MAXWELL, MD, FAAP

pump once a day for 2-3 days, then stop. You might need to pump again in 36-48 hours. If you feel full again after this time, then pump again until you feel comfortable (you won't need to completely drain your breasts).

Be mindful that when you start to decrease the number of pumping sessions, your supply might drastically decrease. Some women have extra bags of frozen milk on standby in case their baby wants more milk during this weaning process.

Even though your body is being told to produce less milk, some women get engorged breasts during the weaning process. You can use cold/frozen cabbage leaves directly on your breasts to relieve the swelling. Keep in mind that some women go through a sort of emotional rollercoaster when weaning their baby. They feel a sense of loss, and that is perfectly normal. It is just an indicator that you are entering a different phase of parenting/motherhood.

CHAPTER 13

When to Supplement

Supplementing can be a contentious topic. First, let me state that if you find that you need to supplement your breastfeeding with donor breast milk or formula, please do not see it as a breastfeeding failure. You have done a great job in providing milk for your baby, and any amount of breast milk is beneficial for your baby! First, talk with a lactation consultant to see if there are other options for increasing your milk supply. Keep in mind that oftentimes when a mother thinks her milk supply is low, it is actually sufficient for her baby.

There are a slew of options available for supplementation. If your child is under 12 months old, they should only supplement with either donor breast milk or formula (per the American Academy of Pediatrics Guidelines).

After that, they can drink any other type of milk (whether it is plant milk or animal milk).

There are several donor milk banks available where you can purchase human milk. If you choose to go this route, only purchase from a milk bank that is HMBANA certified. The milk will likely cost more, but the safety of it is more assured than from other non-HMBANA banks or from group sharing sites. Women who donate breast milk to HMBANA banks undergo a rigorous pre-qualification process where their medical, social, and pregnancy history is taken. If they pass this process, then the mother's blood is tested for infectious diseases, and if the blood cultures are negative, then the milk is defrosted, pooled, pasteurized, and cultured to see if it grows any pathogenic bacteria.

All of these steps are eliminated when you buy milk from a non-HMBANA bank or if you obtain it informally from another mother. That is a risk that some mothers are willing to take. However, there are some babies who have medical conditions in which the safety of their primary diet HAS to be vetted.

Option two is formula. There are many different types available, so I won't go into detail about them here. Some of the main formula companies are Similac, Enfamil, and Gerber. Depending on whether your baby has a milk protein allergy, or if you choose to give a plant-based formula, there are many options from which to choose.

However you choose to supplement, there is one recommendation that I will give—do not mix your expressed breast milk with any other human milk or with formula. Mixing your expressed breast milk with any other type of milk or formula will make it difficult to assess for your baby's tolerance of the new milk.

CHAPTER 14

WHEN TO SEEK
PROFESSIONAL HELP

Believe it or not, quite a few women are not aware of the resources available to them when it comes to help with breastfeeding. Seeking the help of a lactation consultant, even from early on before any problems arise, helps bolster confidence with breastfeeding and can keep you on the alert for any potential issues that may lie ahead. Some women establish a relationship with a lactation consultant before they deliver (prenatally). This can be very important to help address an individual woman's barriers to breastfeeding.

There are many different layers of support available to women, ranging from physicians (pediatrician, OB/GYN, family medicine physician), nurses, lactation consultants, or other allied health professionals. There are several types of breastfeeding support specialists, and they vary simply by the degree of certification that they hold (lactation educators, lactation peer counselors, breastfeeding counselors and lactation consultants). When it comes to lactation consultants, the most "qualified" are IBCLC (International Board Certified Lactation Consultant). Oftentimes, insurance companies will offer coverage for lactation consultants, and some of these will even come directly to your house to help with breastfeeding and provide tips.

Some mothers have also found breastfeeding support groups to be of great help. These can vary from nationwide groups like La Leche League to more informal peer support groups, (including your circle of friends or associates who have breastfed their infant(s).

If your baby has a difficult time latching, becomes frustrated at the breast, or if you feel as if your breasts are not emptied after a breastfeeding session, you should seek help. If your nipples are flattened, there are various devices that can be used to aid the removal of milk while breastfeeding.

CHAPTER 15

REVIEW OF
BREAST PUMPS

There are several breast pumps available on the market. Before purchasing a breast pump, call your health insurance plan to determine if it provides coverage for a breast pump. The best time to call is in your second or third trimester. Your insurance plan will determine what type of breast pump is covered and how you can obtain it.

There are three types of breast pumps—manual, single electric, and double electric. If you plan to use a breast pump occasionally (once or twice a week) and will primarily feed the baby directly from the breast, then a manual breast pump will suffice. If you plan to use the breast pump on a regular basis (for example, you work in the daytime and need to maintain your milk supply while you're away from your baby), then a single or double electric pump will be best. If your infant was born prematurely, is too sick to

breastfeed, has difficulty nursing, or if you are exclusively pumping, have had breast reduction surgery, or have a
medical condition that makes it difficult to produce an
adequate milk supply, then a hospital grade double electric
pump is the best route to go. They can be obtained by your
physician writing a letter of medical necessity on your be-
half. These types of pumps are designed to help a mother
initiate and maintain her milk supply over a longer period
of time.

In addition to considering how often you plan to use
the breast pump, there are additional factors to consider: a
car adaptor if you will be spending time in a car during the
times you usually breastfeed, how easy is it to wash and assemble the pieces of the breast pump (if there are multiple
steps or parts involved, it might become frustrating), how
frequently you plan on using the breast pump (you might
consider looking at more lightweight models), hands-free
option (for those moms who like to multi-task), options
for different flange sizes (the part of the pump that goes
over the breast) depending on the size of your breasts and
nipples and the ability to change the suction to your comfort level. Some pumps have dual phase technology where

they have an initiation/milk letdown phase as well as the regular pumping phase.

The following are some examples of breast pump brands available (This list is not meant to be an exhaustive list. It is merely meant to inform you of available breasts pumps and is not an endorsement of any particular brand).

1. Willow (They specialize in hands-free pumps)
2. Freemie
3. Elvie Pump (currently sold out)
4. The Pump by Babyation (wait list)
5. Medela
6. Hygeia
7. Spectra
8. Lansinoh
9. Ameda
10. BelleMa

CHAPTER 16

SAMPLE SCHEDULE OF WHEN TO PUMP AND ITEMS YOU'LL NEED

When your infant is a newborn, it is important to breast-feed or pump as frequently as possible. This is the stage of your breastfeeding journey where you will initiate and establish your milk supply. Allow your baby to feed on demand at any time. For mothers who opt to exclusively give expressed breast milk, it is just as important to pump frequently, especially in your baby's first 2 months of life. You should pump at least 10-12 times a day for newborns, and then you can decrease the frequency as your infant gets older. Generally, most babies start to sleep for longer stretches of time around 3-4 months, and at this time, you can stop using the breast pump at night. I will include a few sample schedules of when to use the breast pump. You generally want to pump for a minimum of 20 minutes (30 minutes maximum)

Newborn (you want to get in at least 10 sessions minimally, but ideally 12 sessions)

Session 1: 🕐 7am,   Session 2: 🕐 9am,
Session 3: 🕐 11am,   Session 4: 🕐 1pm,
Session 5: 🕐 3pm,   Session 6: 🕐 5pm,
Session 7: 🕐 7pm,   Session 8: 🕐 9pm,
Session 9: 🕐 12am,   Session 10: 🕐 3am,
Session 11: 🕐 5am,   Session 12: 🕐 7 am

Session 2: After about 3-4 weeks, you can pump 8 times in a 24-hour period

Session 1: 🕐 7am,   Session 2: 🕐 10am,
Session 3: 🕐 12pm,   Session 4: 🕐 3pm,
Session 5: 🕐 6pm,   Session 6: 🕐 9pm,
Session 7: 🕐 12am,   Session 8: 🕐 4am

Session 3: Once baby starts to sleep for longer stretches at night (about 6-8 hours at around 3-4 months), you can go down to 6 sessions and eliminate the night sessions

Session 1: 🕐 6am,   Session 2: 🕐 10am,
Session 3: 🕐 12pm,   Session 4: 🕐 3pm,
Session 5: 🕐 6pm,   Session 6: 🕐 10pm

Session 4: By about 5 months, you should be able to decrease to 5 sessions

Session 1: 🕐 6am,   Session 2: 🕚 11am,
Session 3: 🕓 4pm,   Session 4: 🕖 7pm,
Session 5: 🕙 10pm

Personally, once I started to pump less than 5 sessions, my breast milk supply decreased. However, if you have an oversupply and would like to further decrease your pumping frequency, here is a **sample schedule for four sessions:**

Session 1: 🕐 6am,   Session 2: 🕚 11am,
Session 3: 🕓 4pm,   Session 4: 🕘 9pm

The following are a list of suggested items that will make exclusive breast pumping easier:

- [ ] *Extra set of breast pump parts*
- [ ] *Extra bottles (If you can purchase bottles that can attach to your breast pump directly and you can in turn feed directly to your baby, it will be a huge time saver!)*
- [ ] *Breast pads (to avoid your clothes getting wet during random milk letdown)*
- [ ] *Hand-free bra (optional)*
- [ ] *Breast milk freezing/storage bags*
- [ ] *Nursing/breast pumping cover (This is to give you a certain level of privacy while using the breast pump)*
- [ ] *Water bottle and snacks*
- [ ] *Cooler with an ice pack to store milk while away from home*
- [ ] *Dish soap, bottle brush (to clean breast pump parts)*

www.ingramcontent.com/pod-product-compliance
Lightning Source LLC
Chambersburg PA
CBHW030029290326
41934CB00005B/548